HOMESTEAD COOKBOOK

40+Tart, Ice-Cream, and Pie recipes for a healthy and balanced Homestead diet

TABLE OF CONTENTS

equally by a Committee of the American Bar Association and a Committee of Publishers and Associations.

Introduction

Homestead recipes for personal enjoyment but also for family enjoyment. You will love them for sure for how easy it is to prepare them.

ZUCCHINI APPLE PANCAKES

Serves: **4**

Prep Time: **10**   minutes

Cook Time: **10**   minutes

Total Time: **20**   minutes

INGREDIENTS

- 1 zucchini
- 2 tablespoons almond butter
- 2 eggs
- 1 tablespoon honey
- 2 tablespoons coconut oil
- 1 apple
- 1 cup almond flour
- ¼ tsp baking powder
- ¼ tsp sea salt

DIRECTIONS

1. Mix zucchini, honey, apples, thyme and almond butter in a bowl
2. In another bowl mix salt, baking powder and flour and beat the eggs
3. Mix all the ingredients from the bowl and heat coconut oil in a fry pan

4. Pour the mixture in the pan and cook for 1-2 minutes each side

QUINOA AND GOJI BERRIES

Serves: **4**

Prep Time: **5**   Minutes

Cook Time: **10**   Minutes

Total Time: **15**   Minutes

INGREDIENTS

- 1 cup quinoa
- 1 cup goji
- parsley as needed

DIRECTIONS

1. Soak the quinoa and goji grains for 5-6 minutes in water
2. Cook quinoa until soft for 10-15 minutes
3. Roast the cumin seeds in a hot pan and stir in goji berries and sprinkle with parsley

Serves:　　　*2*

Prep Time:　*10*　Minutes

Cook Time:　*20*　Minutes

Total Time:　*30*　Minutes

INGREDIENTS

- 2 cloves garlic
- 2 sausages
- ¼ onion
- ¼ cup carrot
- 2 cups mushrooms
- 1 tsp coconut oil
- ¼ tablespoon parsley
- 2 cups asparagus

DIRECTIONS

1. Sauté the garlic and onions in coconut oil and add the rest of the ingredients
2. Add the sausages and cook for 5-10 minutes, serve when ready

Serves: **3**

Prep Time: **10** Minutes

Cook Time: **10** Minutes

Total Time: **20** Minutes

INGREDIENTS

- 1 cauliflower heat
- 1 tablespoon salt
- 1 tablespoon pepper
- basil
- 1 tablespoon coconut oil
- 1 tablespoon parsley

DIRECTIONS

1. Grate the cauliflower to rice-grain
2. In a pan melt coconut oil add basil and add cauliflower and cook for 5-10 minutes
3. Cook until ready, remove and serve

HOMEMADE GRANOLA

Serves: *2*
Prep Time: *10*   Minutes

Cook Time: *10*   Minutes

Total Time: *20*   Minutes

INGREDIENTS

- ¼ cup pumpkin seeds
- ¼ cup apricots
- 1 cup pecans
- ¼ cup almonds
- 1 cup coconut
- ½ cup coconut oil
- ½ cup honey
- 1 tsp cinnamon
- ¼ tsp nutmeg

DIRECTIONS

1. Preheat the oven to 325 F
2. Combine all the ingredients and toss well
3. Spread the mixture on a baking sheet (grease it with coconut oil) and bake for 10-15 minutes
4. When ready remove from oven and stir apricots
5. Let it cool and serve

FRENCH TOAST

Serves: **2**

Prep Time: **10**   Minutes

Cook Time: **10**   Minutes

Total Time: **20**   Minutes

INGREDIENTS

- 2 eggs
- zest of ½ orange
- butter
- 2 tablespoons milk
- 10 slices fruit bread

DIRECTIONS

1. In a bowl mix eggs, orange zest and eggs, beat the eggs before and mix everything together
2. Place a slice of bread into the mixture to soak
3. Place a pan over medium heat
4. Place the bread slices in the pan and cook for 1-2 minutes on each side
5. Remove and serve with maple syrup

COCONUT OMELETTE

Serves: **4**

Prep Time: **10**   Minutes

Cook Time: **10**   Minutes

Total Time: **20**   Minutes

INGREDIENTS

- 2 eggs
- ½ tsp honey
- 1 tsp coconut oil

DIRECTIONS

1. In a bowl beat 2 eggs, add honey and stir
2. In a frying pan heat coconut oil over medium heat and pour the mixture
3. Cook on each side for 1-2 minutes
4. Remove and serve with salt or pepper

BANANA BREAKFAST CHEESECAKE

Serves: *1*
Prep Time: *10*   Minutes

Cook Time: *10*   Minutes

Total Time: *20*   Minutes

INGREDIENTS

- 2 tsp chocolate chips
- vanilla extract
- 1 tsp almond butter
- 1 tsp honey
- 2 tablespoons oats
- 1 tablespoon cream cheese
- 1 banana

DIRECTIONS

1. In a bowl mix almond butter, oats and honey
2. Slice a banana and add it to the mixture
3. In the microwave add chocolate chips for 1 minute, add vanilla extract and cream cheese to the melted chocolate
4. Top the banana with chocolate mixture and serve

GOJI BERRIES PANCAKES

Serves: **4**

Prep Time: **10** Minutes

Cook Time: **30** Minutes

Total Time: **40** Minutes

INGREDIENTS

- 1 cup whole wheat flour
- ¼ tsp baking soda
- ¼ tsp baking powder
- 2 tablespoons goji berries
- 2 eggs
- 1 cup milk

DIRECTIONS

1. In a bowl combine all ingredients together and mix well
2. In a skillet heat olive oil
3. Pour ¼ of the batter and cook each pancake for 1-2 minutes per side
4. When ready remove from heat and serve

KIWI PANCAKES

Serves: **4**

Prep Time: **10** Minutes

Cook Time: **20** Minutes

Total Time: **30** Minutes

INGREDIENTS

- 1 cup whole wheat flour
- ¼ tsp baking soda
- ¼ tsp baking powder
- 1 cup mashed kiwi
- 2 eggs
- 1 cup milk

DIRECTIONS

1. In a bowl combine all ingredients together and mix well
2. In a skillet heat olive oil
3. Pour ¼ of the batter and cook each pancake for 1-2 minutes per side
4. When ready remove from heat and serve

MANGO PANCAKES

Serves: **4**

Prep Time: **10**   Minutes

Cook Time: **20**   Minutes

Total Time: **30**   Minutes

INGREDIENTS

- 1 cup whole wheat flour
- ¼ tsp baking soda
- ¼ tsp baking powder
- 1 cup mashed mango
- 2 eggs
- 1 cup milk

DIRECTIONS

1. In a bowl combine all ingredients together and mix well
2. In a skillet heat olive oil
3. Pour ¼ of the batter and cook each pancake for 1-2 minutes per side
4. When ready remove from heat and serve

SIMPLE PANCAKES

Serves: **4**

Prep Time: **10** Minutes

Cook Time: **30** Minutes

Total Time: **40** Minutes

INGREDIENTS

- 1 cup whole wheat flour
- ¼ tsp baking soda
- ¼ tsp baking powder
- 2 eggs
- 1 cup milk

DIRECTIONS

1. In a bowl combine all ingredients together and mix well
2. In a skillet heat olive oil
3. Pour ¼ of the batter and cook each pancake for 1-2 minutes per side
4. When ready remove from heat and serve

GINGERBREAD MUFFINS

Serves:	*8-12*
Prep Time:	**10** Minutes
Cook Time:	**20** Minutes
Total Time:	**30** Minutes

INGREDIENTS

- 2 eggs
- 1 tablespoon olive oil
- 1 cup milk
- 2 cups whole wheat flour
- 1 tsp baking soda
- ¼ tsp baking soda
- 1 tsp ginger
- 1 tsp cinnamon
- ¼ cup molasses

DIRECTIONS

1. In a bowl combine all dry ingredients
2. In another bowl combine all dry ingredients
3. Combine wet and dry ingredients together
4. Fold in ginger and mix well
5. Pour mixture into 8-12 prepared muffin cups, fill 2/3 of the cups

6. Bake for 18-20 minutes at 375 F
7. When ready remove from the oven and serve

PEAR MUFFINS

Serves: **8-12**

Prep Time: **10**   Minutes

Cook Time: **20**   Minutes

Total Time: **30**   Minutes

INGREDIENTS

- 2 eggs
- 1 tablespoon olive oil
- 1 cup milk
- 2 cups whole wheat flour
- 1 tsp baking soda
- ¼ tsp baking soda
- 1 tsp cinnamon
- 1 cup mashed pear

DIRECTIONS

1. In a bowl combine all dry ingredients
2. In another bowl combine all dry ingredients
3. Combine wet and dry ingredients together
4. Pour mixture into 8-12 prepared muffin cups, fill 2/3 of the cups
5. Bake for 18-20 minutes at 375 F
6. When ready remove from the oven and serve

POMELO MUFFINS

Serves: **8-12**
Prep Time: **10**   Minutes

Cook Time: **20**   Minutes

Total Time: **30**   Minutes

INGREDIENTS

- 2 eggs
- 1 tablespoon olive oil
- 1 cup milk
- 2 cups whole wheat flour
- 1 tsp baking soda
- ¼ tsp baking soda
- 1 tsp cinnamon
- 1 cup pomelo

DIRECTIONS

1. In a bowl combine all dry ingredients
2. In another bowl combine all dry ingredients
3. Combine wet and dry ingredients together
4. Pour mixture into 8-12 prepared muffin cups, fill 2/3 of the cups
5. Bake for 18-20 minutes at 375 F
6. When ready remove from the oven and serve

APPLE MUFFINS

Serves: *8-12*

Prep Time: *10* Minutes

Cook Time: *20* Minutes

Total Time: *30* Minutes

INGREDIENTS

- 2 eggs
- 1 tablespoon olive oil
- 1 cup milk
- 2 cups whole wheat flour
- 1 tsp baking soda
- ¼ tsp baking soda
- 1 tsp cinnamon
- 1 cup apple

DIRECTIONS

1. In a bowl combine all dry ingredients
2. In another bowl combine all dry ingredients
3. Combine wet and dry ingredients together
4. Pour mixture into 8-12 prepared muffin cups, fill 2/3 of the cups
5. Bake for 18-20 minutes at 375 F
6. When ready remove from the oven and serve

CHOCOLATE MUFFINS

Serves: **8-12**

Prep Time: **10**   Minutes

Cook Time: **20**   Minutes

Total Time: **30**   Minutes

INGREDIENTS

- 2 eggs
- 1 tablespoon olive oil
- 1 cup milk
- 2 cups whole wheat flour
- 1 tsp baking soda
- ¼ tsp baking soda
- 1 tsp cinnamon
- 1 cup chocolate chips

DIRECTIONS

1. In a bowl combine all dry ingredients
2. In another bowl combine all dry ingredients
3. Combine wet and dry ingredients together
4. Fold in chocolate chips and mix well
5. Pour mixture into 8-12 prepared muffin cups, fill 2/3 of the cups
6. Bake for 18-20 minutes at 375 F

7. When ready remove from the oven and serve

SIMPLE MUFFINS

Serves: *8-12*

Prep Time: *10*   Minutes

Cook Time: *20*   Minutes

Total Time: *30*   Minutes

INGREDIENTS

- 2 eggs
- 1 tablespoon olive oil
- 1 cup milk
- 2 cups whole wheat flour
- 1 tsp baking soda
- ¼ tsp baking soda
- 1 tsp cinnamon

DIRECTIONS

1. In a bowl combine all dry ingredients
2. In another bowl combine all dry ingredients
3. Combine wet and dry ingredients together
4. Pour mixture into 8-12 prepared muffin cups, fill 2/3 of the cups
5. Bake for 18-20 minutes at 375 F
6. When ready remove from the oven and serve

SPINACH OMELETTE

Serves: **1**

Prep Time: **5**   Minutes

Cook Time: **10**   Minutes

Total Time: **15**   Minutes

INGREDIENTS

- 2 eggs
- ¼ tsp salt
- ¼ tsp black pepper
- 1 tablespoon olive oil
- ¼ cup cheese
- ¼ tsp basil
- 1 cup spinach

DIRECTIONS

1. In a bowl combine all ingredients together and mix well
2. In a skillet heat olive oil and pour the egg mixture
3. Cook for 1-2 minutes per side
4. When ready remove omelette from the skillet and serve

CUCUMBER OMELETTE

Serves: **1**

Prep Time: **5**   Minutes

Cook Time: **10**   Minutes

Total Time: **15**   Minutes

INGREDIENTS

- 2 eggs
- ¼ tsp salt
- ¼ tsp black pepper
- 1 tablespoon olive oil
- ¼ cup cheese
- ¼ tsp basil
- ½ cup cucumber

DIRECTIONS

1. In a bowl combine all ingredients together and mix well
2. In a skillet heat olive oil and pour the egg mixture
3. Cook for 1-2 minutes per side
4. When ready remove omelette from the skillet and serve

BASIL OMELETTE

Serves: *1*
Prep Time: 5   Minutes

Cook Time: *10*   Minutes

Total Time: *15*   Minutes

INGREDIENTS

- 2 eggs
- ¼ tsp salt
- ¼ tsp black pepper
- 1 tablespoon olive oil
- ¼ cup cheese
- ¼ tsp basil
- 1 cup red onion

DIRECTIONS

1. In a bowl combine all ingredients together and mix well
2. In a skillet heat olive oil and pour the egg mixture
3. Cook for 1-2 minutes per side
4. When ready remove omelette from the skillet and serve

CHEESE OMELETTE

Serves: **1**

Prep Time: **5** Minutes

Cook Time: **10** Minutes

Total Time: **15** Minutes

INGREDIENTS

- 2 eggs
- ¼ tsp salt
- ¼ tsp black pepper
- 1 tablespoon olive oil
- ¼ cup cheese
- ¼ tsp basil
- 1 cup mushrooms

DIRECTIONS

1. In a bowl combine all ingredients together and mix well
2. In a skillet heat olive oil and pour the egg mixture
3. Cook for 1-2 minutes per side
4. When ready remove omelette from the skillet and serve

OLIVE OMELETTE

Serves: **1**

Prep Time: **5**   Minutes

Cook Time: **10**   Minutes

Total Time: **15**   Minutes

INGREDIENTS

- 2 eggs
- ¼ tsp salt
- ¼ tsp black pepper
- 1 tablespoon olive oil
- ¼ cup cheese
- ¼ cup Kalamata olives
- ¼ tsp basil
- 1 cup tomatoes

DIRECTIONS

1. In a bowl combine all ingredients together and mix well
2. In a skillet heat olive oil and pour the egg mixture
3. Cook for 1-2 minutes per side
4. When ready remove omelette from the skillet and serve

CARDAMOM TART

Serves: **6-8**

Prep Time: **25**   Minutes

Cook Time: **25**   Minutes

Total Time: **50**   Minutes

INGREDIENTS

- 4-5 pears
- 2 tablespoons lemon juice
- pastry sheets

CARDAMOM FILLING

- ½ lb. butter
- ½ lb. brown sugar
- ½ lb. almonds
- ¼ lb. flour
- 1 ¼ tsp cardamom
- 2 eggs

DIRECTIONS

1. Preheat oven to 400 F, unfold pastry sheets and place them on a baking sheet
2. Toss together all ingredients together and mix well

3. Spread mixture in a single layer on the pastry sheets
4. Before baking decorate with your desired fruits
5. Bake at 400 F for 22-25 minutes or until golden brown
6. When ready remove from the oven and serve

APPLE TART

Serves: *6-8*
Prep Time: *25*   Minutes

Cook Time: *25*   Minutes

Total Time: *50*   Minutes

INGREDIENTS

- pastry sheets

FILLING

- 1 tsp lemon juice
- 3 oz. brown sugar
- 1 lb. apples
- 150 ml double cream
- 2 eggs

DIRECTIONS

1. Preheat oven to 400 F, unfold pastry sheets and place them on a baking sheet
2. Toss together all ingredients together and mix well
3. Spread mixture in a single layer on the pastry sheets
4. Before baking decorate with your desired fruits
5. Bake at 400 F for 22-25 minutes or until golden brown
6. When ready remove from the oven and serve

PEACH PECAN PIE

Serves: *8-12*

Prep Time: *15*   Minutes

Cook Time: *35*   Minutes

Total Time: *50*   Minutes

INGREDIENTS

- 4-5 cups peaches
- 1 tablespoon preserves
- 1 cup sugar
- 4 small egg yolks
- ¼ cup flour
- 1 tsp vanilla extract

DIRECTIONS

1. Line a pie plate or pie form with pastry and cover the edges of the plate depending on your preference
2. In a bowl combine all pie ingredients together and mix well
3. Pour the mixture over the pastry
4. Bake at 400-425 F for 25-30 minutes or until golden brown
5. When ready remove from the oven and let it rest for 15 minutes

GRAPEFRUIT PIE

Serves: *8-12*

Prep Time: *15*   Minutes

Cook Time: *35*   Minutes

Total Time: *50*   Minutes

INGREDIENTS

- pastry sheets
- 2 cups grapefruit
- 1 cup brown sugar
- ¼ cup flour
- 5-6 egg yolks
- 5 oz. butter

DIRECTIONS

1. Line a pie plate or pie form with pastry and cover the edges of the plate depending on your preference
2. In a bowl combine all pie ingredients together and mix well
3. Pour the mixture over the pastry
4. Bake at 400-425 F for 25-30 minutes or until golden brown
5. When ready remove from the oven and let it rest for 15 minutes

BUTTERFINGER PIE

Serves: **8-12**

Prep Time: **15** Minutes

Cook Time: **35** Minutes

Total Time: **50** Minutes

INGREDIENTS

- pastry sheets
- 1 package cream cheese
- 1 tsp vanilla extract
- ¼ cup peanut butter
- 1 cup powdered sugar (to decorate)
- 2 cups Butterfinger candy bars
- 8 oz whipped topping

DIRECTIONS

1. Line a pie plate or pie form with pastry and cover the edges of the plate depending on your preference
2. In a bowl combine all pie ingredients together and mix well
3. Pour the mixture over the pastry
4. Bake at 400-425 F for 25-30 minutes or until golden brown
5. When ready remove from the oven and let it rest for 15 minutes

SMOOTHIE RECIPES

BANANA MATCHA SMOOTHIE

Serves: **1**

Prep Time: **5**   Minutes

Cook Time: **5**   Minutes

Total Time: **10**   Minutes

INGREDIENTS

- 1 cup banana
- 1 tsp matcha powder
- 1 cup spinach
- 1 tsp flax seed
- 1 tsp vanilla extract
- 1 cup soy milk

DIRECTIONS

1. In a blender place all ingredients and blend until smooth
2. Pour smoothie in a glass and serve

Serves: **1**

Prep Time: **5** Minutes

Cook Time: **5** Minutes

Total Time: **10** Minutes

INGREDIENTS

- 2 bananas
- 2 dates
- 1 cup kale
- 1 cup spinach
- 2 tablespoons cocoa powder
- 1 tsp vanilla extract
- 1 cup nut milk

DIRECTIONS

1. In a blender place all ingredients and blend until smooth
2. Pour smoothie in a glass and serve

CREAMY SMOOTHIE

Serves: **1**

Prep Time: 5   Minutes

Cook Time: 5   Minutes

Total Time: **10** Minutes

INGREDIENTS

- 1 cup strawberries
- 1 banana
- 1 cup Greek Yogurt
- 1 cup soy milk
- 1 tsp vanilla extract
- 1 tsp chia seeds

DIRECTIONS

1. In a blender place all ingredients and blend until smooth
2. Pour smoothie in a glass and serve

Serves: **1**

Prep Time: 5 Minutes

Cook Time: 5 Minutes

Total Time: **10** Minutes

INGREDIENTS

- 1 cup strawberries
- 1 banana
- 1 cup Greek Yogurt
- 1 scoop protein powder
- 1 tsp hemp seeds
- ½ cup chocolate chips

DIRECTIONS

1. In a blender place all ingredients and blend until smooth
2. Pour smoothie in a glass and serve

APPLE SMOOTHIE

Serves: **1**

Prep Time: **5**   Minutes

Cook Time: **5**   Minutes

Total Time: **10**   Minutes

INGREDIENTS

- 1 apple
- 2 pears
- ½ cup rolled oats
- 1 tsp cinnamon
- 1 cup nut milk

DIRECTIONS

1. In a blender place all ingredients and blend until smooth
2. Pour smoothie in a glass and serve

SPINACH SMOOTHIE

Serves: *1*

Prep Time: 5   Minutes

Cook Time: 5   Minutes

Total Time: *10*   Minutes

INGREDIENTS

- 1 banana
- 1 cup vanilla yogurt
- 1 cup spinach
- 1 cup kale
- 1 cup orange juice

DIRECTIONS

1. In a blender place all ingredients and blend until smooth
2. Pour smoothie in a glass and serve

PEANUT BUTTER SMOOTHIE

Serves: **1**

Prep Time: **5** Minutes

Cook Time: **5** Minutes

Total Time: **10** Minutes

INGREDIENTS

- 1 cup berries
- 2 tablespoons peanut butter
- ½ cup protein powder
- ½ cup oats
- 1 cup soy milk

DIRECTIONS

1. In a blender place all ingredients and blend until smooth
2. Pour smoothie in a glass and serve

PINEAPPLE SMOOTHIE

Serves: **1**

Prep Time: **5**   Minutes

Cook Time: **5**   Minutes

Total Time: **10**   Minutes

INGREDIENTS

- 1 cup pineapple
- 1 cup strawberries
- 1 cup Greek yogurt
- 1 cup soy milk
- 1 cup ice

DIRECTIONS

1. In a blender place all ingredients and blend until smooth
2. Pour smoothie in a glass and serve

ORANGE SMOOTHIE

Serves: **1**
Prep Time: 5   Minutes

Cook Time: 5   Minutes

Total Time: **10**   Minutes

INGREDIENTS

- 1 orange
- ½ cup orange juice
- ½ banana
- 1 tsp vanilla essence

DIRECTIONS

1. In a blender place all ingredients and blend until smooth
2. Pour smoothie in a glass and serve

Serves: **1**

Prep Time: 5   Minutes

Cook Time: 5   Minutes

Total Time: **10**   Minutes

INGREDIENTS

- ¼ cup raisins
- 2 Medjool dates
- 1 cup berries
- 1 cup almond milk
- 1 tsp chia seeds

DIRECTIONS

1. In a blender place all ingredients and blend until smooth
2. Pour smoothie in a glass and serve

ICE-CREAM RECIPES

PISTACHIOS ICE-CREAM

Serves: *6-8*

Prep Time: *15*   Minutes
Cook Time: *15*   Minutes
Total Time: *30*   Minutes

INGREDIENTS

- 4 egg yolks
- 1 cup heavy cream
- 1 cup milk
- 1 cup sugar
- 1 vanilla bean
- 1 tsp almond extract
- 1 cup cherries
- ½ cup pistachios

DIRECTIONS

1. In a saucepan whisk together all ingredients
2. Mix until bubbly
3. Strain into a bowl and cool
4. Whisk in favorite fruits and mix well
5. Cover and refrigerate for 2-3 hours

6. Pour mixture in the ice-cream maker and follow manufacturer instructions

7. Serve when ready

VANILLA ICE-CREAM

Serves: **6-8**

Prep Time: **15**   Minutes
Cook Time: **15**   Minutes
Total Time: **30**   Minutes

INGREDIENTS

- 1 cup milk
- 1 tablespoon cornstarch
- 1 oz. cream cheese
- 1 cup heavy cream
- 1 cup brown sugar
- 1 tablespoon corn syrup
- 1 vanilla bean

DIRECTIONS

1. In a saucepan whisk together all ingredients
2. Mix until bubbly
3. Strain into a bowl and cool
4. Whisk in favorite fruits and mix well
5. Cover and refrigerate for 2-3 hours
6. Pour mixture in the ice-cream maker and follow manufacturer instructions
7. Serve when ready

COFFE ICE-CREAM

Serves: *6-8*

Prep Time: *15*   Minutes

Cook Time: *15*   Minutes

Total Time: *30*   Minutes

INGREDIENTS

- 4 egg yolks
- 1 cup black coffee
- 2 cups heavy cream
- 1 cup half-and-half
- 1 cup brown sugar
- 1 tsp vanilla extract

DIRECTIONS

1. In a saucepan whisk together all ingredients
2. Mix until bubbly
3. Strain into a bowl and cool
4. Whisk in favorite fruits and mix well
5. Cover and refrigerate for 2-3 hours
6. Pour mixture in the ice-cream maker and follow manufacturer instructions
7. Serve when ready

THANK YOU FOR READING THIS BOOK!

CPSIA information can be obtained
at www.ICGtesting.com
Printed in the USA
BVHW031359150321
602550BV00001B/382

9 781664 047204